The Low Carb Bible

The Low Carb Cookbook with Quick and Easy Recipes
incl. 10 Steps to Lose Weight Fast

[1st Edition]

James Anthony Brooks

Copyright © [2019] [James Anthony Brooks]

Alle Rechte vorbehalten

Die Rechte des hier dargestellten Buches liegen ausschließlich beim Verfasser.
Eine Verwendung und Verarbeitung des Textes ist untersagt und bedarf in
Ausnahmefällen einer klaren Zustimmung des Verfassers.

ISBN: 9781693528361

Table of Contents

Introduction... 1

    What is Low Carb?..2

    History of Low Carb 3

    Everything You Need to Know About Carbs..3

What Happens in Our Body? 5

    Used for Fuel 5

    Saved for Later 6

    Stored as Fat 6

Is Low Carb Really Healthy? 7

    Decrease Overall Appetite 7

    More Weight Loss at First 8

    More Fat is Lost from Abdomen Area 8

    Drastic Reduction in Triglycerides...9

    "Good" HDL Cholesterol Increases 9

    "Bad" LDL Cholesterol Decreases 9

    Reduction in Insulin and Blood Sugar Levels 10

Decrease Blood Pressure 10

Treats Several Brain Disorders 11

What Should I Avoid? **12**

Breads/Grains 12

Some Fruits 13

Starchy Veggies 14

Pasta 14

Breakfast Cereal 15

Beer 15

Sweetened Yogurt 16

Juice 16

Low-Fat/Fat-Free Salad Dressings 17

Beans/Legumes 17

Honey/Sugar (any kind) 18

Chips/Crackers 18

Milk 19

Gluten-Free Baked Goods 19

What am I Allowed to Eat? **21**

Meat 21

Fish/Seafood 21

Eggs 22

Natural Fats/High-Fat Sauces 22

Veggies 22

Dairy 22

Nuts 23

Berries 23

Drinks 23

Celebrations/Special Events 23

How Many Carbs Should I Consume Each Day? 25

How to Get Started on a Low Carb Eating Plan 27

Reduce Carb Consumption 28

Stay Full & Satisfied 30

Choose a Diet You Can Stick With Long-Term 31

Atkins.. 31

South Beach Diet 32

Ketogenic Diet 32

Dukan Diet 33

Paleo Diet 33

Stay Healthy & Motivated 34

Low Carb Recipes 36

Low Carb Breakfast Recipes 37

Goat Cheese & Herb Omelet.. 38

Frittata with Spinach & Goat Cheese.. 39

Fried Egg Sandwich 40

Spinach Quiche (No Crust) 41

Egg & Cheese Boats.. 42

Sausage Casserole.. 43

Oven Scrambled Eggs...44

Oven-Baked Denver Omelet 45

Ham, Cheese, & Hashbrown Casserole..46

French Toast..47

Low Carb Lunch Recipes **48**

Chipped Beef on Toast 49

Low Carb Burger...50

Beef Dip Sandwich..51

Garlic Salmon 52

Bacon & Feta Stuffed Chicken Breasts 53

Turkey Burgers with Feta Cheese..54

Ham & Cheese Rolls...55

BBQ Bacon Shrimp...56

Grilled Mushrooms 57

Grilled Tandoori Chicken..58

Meatballs w/ Sweet & Sour Sauce...59

Herby Lemon Chicken...60

Gyro Burger...61

Low Carb Dinner Recipes... **62**

Lasagna Stuffed Peppers 63

Chicken Cacciatore...64

Roast Chicken w/ Lemon & Carrots 65

Stuffed Summer Squash 66

Candied Bacon Chicken with Cauliflower Rice & Pecans........................67

Lettuce Wraps...69

Beef Slaw...70

Lasagna Stuffed Mushrooms 71

Sweet Potato Carbonara with Mushrooms & Spinach.........................72

Grilled Salmon Wraps..73

Parmesan Tilapia..74

Pork Chops with Mushroom Sauce 75

Low Carb Dessert Recipes **76**

Almond-Raspberry Cupcakes..77

Chocolate-Peanut Butter Whip...78

Pumpkin Pecan Cheesecake..79

Vanilla Almond Butter Cookies...81

Tiramisu Cupcakes 82

Low Carb Snack Recipes **84**

Blackberry-Coconut Fat Bombs..85

Pizza Bites...86

Salt & Vinegar Zucchini Chips...87

Chocolate Quinoa Bites...88

Pepper Nachos 89

Low Carb Smoothie Recipes **90**

Chocolate-Avocado Smoothie...91

Very Berry Smoothie 92

Chocolate Peanut Butter Smoothie..93

Coffee Smoothie...94

Avocado/Spinach/Strawberry Smoothie..95

Bonus: 10 Ways to Lose Weight Fast **96**

Begin Your Day with Warm Lemon Water 96

Get at least 30 mins of Physical Activity Daily 96

Be Sure to Get Your Fiber 97

Consume Healthy Protein Sources at Every Meal 97

Pay Attention to What You're Eating 97

Choose Healthy Snacks 97

Discover Healthy Alternatives to Your Favorite Treats 98

Learn to Manage Your Stress 98

Kick Those Bad Habits 98

Make a Plan to be Successful 98

Disclaimer **100**

Introduction

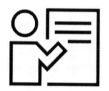

Chances are, you've heard the term "low carb" at some point. In fact, lately, it's become one of the diet buzzwords that everyone seems to be talking about. However, have you ever wondered what it really means? Let's take a look:

What is Low Carb?

Carbs- such as flour and white sugar- while they may taste great, can result in a variety of health issues, including sugar imbalances. However, you can kickstart your body's' metabolism by decreasing the amount of carbs you consume. This encourages your body to burn excess fat for energy.

When you consume carbs, they are converted into glucose, which will remain provide your body with a quick energy boost. If not used right away, your body will store the glycogen in your liver and muscles to be used later. If you consume excess carbs that your body really doesn't need, they are converted into fat. Later, when you consume more carbs, your body uses those instead of tapping into your fat stores. You may not know it, but if your diet is rich in carbs, your body will just keep using those- and storing what it doesn't need at the moment. This causes your body's natural fat-burning process to shut down.

The worst part about it is, since your body easily digests carbs, they don't really do much to stop hunger pangs. Therefore, shortly after you eat a meal high in carbs, you'll be hungry again- craving more carbs. Proteins and fats take longer to digest, which means you don't get as hungry as often. Additionally, when you decrease your consumption of "bad" carbs, your glucose levels stabilize, so your energy levels stay pretty stable instead of spiking and dipping all the time. When your blood sugar levels are stable, your body doesn't produce as much insulin (aka, the "fat storage" hormone), which also means you don't experience as many hunger pangs.

Unfortunately, most diets are really only beneficial in the short term and are difficult to maintain because you are restricting your fat and calories, which means you feel hungry all the time. However, when done properly, a low-carb diet is a great approach to eating. In fact, some individuals have reported improvements in medical conditions such as PCOS, epilepsy, and diabetes. Of course, please don't just take our word for it. If you have been diagnosed with a serious medical condition, you should speak with your physician before making any significant changes to your diet.

History of Low Carb

While it's true that low carb diets are really just making headlines, many people have depended upon them for some time due to their health and weight loss benefits. In fact, William Banting, a British undertaker in the Victorian Era who was obese, spoke with several medical specialists to try to get some help with weight loss. Eventually, an ear specialist suggested a radical diet that would limit his consumption of carbs, especially things such as sugar, butter, bread, milk, and potatoes (which were dietary staples of that time). This new way of eating helped him lose a lot of weight, as well as helped give him some relief from many of the ailments that accompanied his obesity.

Now that you have some of the history behind the low-carb way of life, let's look at some things you need to know about carbs.

Everything You Need to Know About Carbs

The very first thing you need to know is this: what is a carbohydrate? A carbohydrate is any large group of starches, cellulose/gums, and sugars that are alike because they are made up of oxygen, hydrogen, and carbon in similar quantities. Your body uses carbs by processing them and turning them into glucose, which is a simple sugar, to fuel it. Typically, 1 g carb is 4 calories.

Now that you know what is meant by the term "carb", you need to know more about what foods contain carbs. You will find simple carbs/simple sugars in refined/processed sugars such as honey, candy, and table sugar- in addition to fruits, veggies, and milk products. Your body will have an easier time digesting simple carbs over complex carbs.

On the other hand, a complex carb is a long chain of simple carbs and are made of starch and fiber. Foods that contain complex carbs encompass starchy veggies- such as potatoes, bread, pasta, cereals, and rice.

You're probably wondering now if that means that some carbs are better/healthier than others. The truth is, when you start a low-carb diet, it's ideal to eliminate them from your diet. However, since complex carbs contain other nutrients, they are better for you than simple carbs. Still, when comparing sugars based on their health value, an apple isn't any better than honey or table sugar. Regardless of the source, your body processes sugar the exact same way.

According to nutritionists, around 55-60% of your daily caloric intake should be from carbs. That's right, when eaten in moderation, carbs are really not all that bad for you. One FDA report revealed what when you consume sugar in moderate quantities, it can't be linked to dependency or any medical conditions. Of course, if you consume too much sugar, you may develop cavities and become obese. However, scientists have not linked sugar to hyperactivity and, in fact, have suggested that sugar may actually be calming for both adults and children.

What Happens in Our Body?

As you've learned, most carbs are made up of large chains of sugar molecules. Before these chains can be absorbed into your blood and used, your body must break them down through the process of digestion.

This process begins in your mouth, where salivary amylase enzymes break down starches (the sugars that exist in potatoes and grains) into smaller molecules. After that, carbs go through your stomach basically unchanged and into your small intestine. At that point, the enzymes in your small intestine will convert the carbs into simple sugars (glucose & fructose). Then, the sugars can go into your bloodstream and be used by your body. They will either be: used for fuel, saved for later, or stored as fat.

Used for Fuel

When it comes to energy, carbs are the body's primary source. Sure, it's true that your body can use fat and protein as energy- after the carb portion of your meal has been burned. Carbs travel through your bloodstream in the form of fructose and glucose and your bodily tissues absorb them.

Your body is able to freely absorb fructose- but needs insulin to absorb glucose. The insulin drives the glucose into your muscles so that they can contract. Once the glucose and fructose have absorbed into your cells, they combine with oxygen to create adenosine triphosphate (ATP)- which is the currency your cells use for energy.

Saved for Later

Once your energy requirements have been met, the remaining carbs will travel to your muscles and liver. At that point, the body will convert it into glycogen, which is a long chain of glucose molecules. Glycogen is a stored form of energy that your body can use to meet energy requirements between your meals or when you're fasting. Your body uses glycogen to balance your glucose levels and help you avoid experiencing hypoglycemia.

Stored as Fat

According to the experts, about 500 grams of glycogen is stored in your muscles and liver. This is equal to 2,000 calories, which can meet the energy requirements of your body for around 18 hours. Any carbs that are not needed for this glycogen storage will then be converted into fatty acids, which your body stores in fat cells as triglycerides. The triglycerides are a concentrated energy source- but your body will only burn them once the glycogen has been depleted. This mechanism was evolved by the human body to protect us against long fasting periods. However, in modern society, fasting/depriving your body of calories is typically done on purpose- known as dieting.

Is Low Carb Really Healthy?

For many years, low carb diets have been the subject of controversy. Some people hold the belief that low-carb diets actually cause your cholesterol to increase and could lead to heart disease. After all, they do typically encourage high fat consumption. The scientific community has actually proven that low-carb diets/lifestyles are actually quite beneficial and healthy. Experts say that low-carb diets will encourage weight loss and improve risk factors for heart disease.

In this section, we're going to explore a few of the health benefits of low-carb diets.

Decrease Overall Appetite

One of the worst side effects of dieting is hunger and is one of the primary reasons that most people are miserable and end up giving up on their diet. Experts say that low-carb dieting automatically reduces your overall appetite because when people cut carbs and increase their consumption of fat and protein, they are not eating nearly as many calories.

More Weight Loss at First

One of the most effective- and simplest- ways to drop a few pounds is to cut carbs. Studies have proven that individuals who go reduce their carb consumption will actually lose weight quickly than those who reduce fact consumption, even though individuals on low fat diets restricting the number of calories they consume.

This is because a low-carb diet actually gets rid of the water weight, which decreases your insulin levels and causes you to lose weight quickly at first. There are some studies that indicate that those who restrict their carb consumption will lose 2-3 times as much weight- and don't' feel like they're starving themselves.

One particular study showed that a low carb diet was especially effective for the first six months when compared with conventional weight loss methods. However, after that, there wasn't a significant difference between the various methods.

More Fat is Lost from Abdomen Area

One thing you need to know is that the fat in your body is not all the same. The way it affects your overall health and risk factors for various medical conditions depends on where it is stored in your body. Fat is categorized into two main types:

- Subcutaneous: under the skin
- Visceral: abdominal area

Visceral fat typically is found surrounding your organs. This type of fat has been associated with inflammation and insulin resistance and could be the driving force behind metabolic dysfunction.

Experts are quick to point out that most people who lose weight on a low carb diet seem to lose it from their abdominal area. Eventually, this could result in a decreased risk of heart disease and type 2 diabetes.

Drastic Reduction in Triglycerides

Triglycerides are the fat molecules that circulate through your bloodstream. Experts have determined that high triglyceride levels after an overnight fast increase your risk of heart disease. Sedentary individuals typically have high triglyceride levels because of their carb consumption.

However, when you start cutting carbs, you're likely to experience a significant reduction in triglycerides in your blood. However, if you consume a low-fat diet, you are more likely to experience the opposite: an increase in triglycerides in the blood.

"Good" HDL Cholesterol Increases

HDL, or high-density lipoprotein- cholesterol is often referred to as "good" cholesterol. The higher your HDL compared to LDL ("bad" cholesterol), the lower your risk of heart disease. One way to increase your HDL cholesterol levels is to consume fat- which is a major component of low-carb diets. Therefore, it's obvious that your HDL will increase on a low-carb diet, while it will only slightly increase or possibly decline on a low-fat diet.

"Bad" LDL Cholesterol Decreases

In addition to increasing your HDL, a low-carb diet also decreases your LDL cholesterol. LDL is known as "bad" cholesterol and contributes to heart disease. Individuals who have elevated LDL levels are more likely to experience a heart attack.

Experts say that in this case, size matters, small LDL particles indicate an increased risk of heart disease, while large ones indicate a decreased risk. The low-carb way of life will decrease the number of LDL particles in your blood and make them bigger.

Therefore, since decreasing your carb consumption increases HDL and decreases LDL, it's actually a great diet for your overall heart health.

Reduction in Insulin and Blood Sugar Levels

Some experts say that low-carb diets are beneficial for those who have insulin resistance and diabetes, which affects millions of people across the world. Studies have revealed that cutting carbs drastically decreases insulin and blood sugar levels. In fact, some individuals with diabetes have claimed that after beginning a low-carb diet, they were able to decrease their insulin dosage by half. In one study of individuals with type 2 diabetes showed that those who started a low-carb diet were able to eliminate (or at least decrease) their medication within 6 months.

Of course, if your physician has prescribed medication to regulate your blood sugar, you'll need to discuss any changes in your diet with him/her. You may need to make adjustments to your medication to avoid hypoglycemia.

Decrease Blood Pressure

One risk factor for several medical conditions is high blood pressure/hypertension. According to the experts, a low carb diet is quite effective for lowering blood pressure, which will decrease your risk of these- and therefore, lead to a longer life.

Treats Several Brain Disorders

Some areas of your brain are powered only by glucose, which is the reason your liver produces it from protein when you're limiting/eliminating carbs from your diet. However, much of your brain also burns ketones, which your body produces during periods of starvation or when you are limiting carbs. This is the point of the ketogenic diet. Professionals have used it for years to treat children with epilepsy that have not responded to medication.

There are many cases in which children on this diet have been cured of epilepsy. One study showed children on this carb-limiting diet had a 50% reduction in the number of seizures they experienced, and 16% of them experienced no seizures. Medical experts are considering low-carb diets as a treatment for other brain conditions, such as Parkinson's and Alzheimer's.

What it comes down to is this: there are very few things that have as many health benefits as the low-carb diet. This lifestyle will have many positive impacts on your overall health, such as:

· Decreasing your appetite

· Lowering triglycerides

· Increase weight loss

· Improved blood sugar, cholesterol, and blood pressure

If you believe that this type of diet is a good idea for you, make sure that you take the time to speak with your physician before taking drastic measures.

What Should I Avoid?

When you set out on a low carb eating plan, it's obvious that foods such as candy, cakes, and sugary sweet drinks should be avoided. However, when it comes to figuring out which staple foods you need to be limiting or avoiding, it can be a bit more challenging. The truth is that some of these are actually healthy, just not great for those on a low-carb eating plan.

Your target daily carb count will determine whether you should completely eliminate these foods or just limit them. Typically, a low carb diet consists of 20 to 100 grams of carbs daily. Following, you'll find 14 foods that you should avoid (or at least limit) when you get started on your low carb diet.

Breads/Grains

Bread comes in a variety of forms, such as tortillas, bagels, rolls, loaves, and flatbreads- and in many cultures, is a staple food. Unfortunately, they're all high in carbs- whether they are made from refined flour or whole-grains. While it's true that the actual carb count will depend upon the portion sizes and ingredients, following are the average carb counts for breads:

- 1 slice white bread: 14 g carbs/1 g is fiber
- 1 slice whole wheat bread: 17 g carbs/2 g is fiber
- 10-in flour tortilla: 36 g carbs/2 g is fiber
- 3-in bagel: 29 g carbs/1 g is fiber

As you can see, depending upon your limits, eating a sandwich, bagel, or burrito could cause you to reach- if not exceed it. In addition, most grains including oats, wheat, and rice have high carb counts and must be limited or avoided on a low carb diet.

Some Fruits

One important fact to note is that eating lots of fruits and veggies has proven to decrease an individual's risk of heart disease and some cancers. On the other hand, many fruits have lots of carbs and are not great for the low-carb dieter. Please note: a typical serving of fruit is 1 cup/120 grams or 1 small piece. For example, one small apple contains 21 g carbs, 4 g are from fiber. Therefore, if you're on a low carb diet, it's probably best to avoid some fruits, especially those that are really sweet and dried, which have higher carb counts.

Following are a few fruits with their carb counts:

- 1 medium banana: 27 g carbs/3 g from fiber
- 1 oz/28 g raisins: 22 g carbs/1 g from fiber
- 2 large dates: 36 g carbs/4 g from fiber
- 1 cup/165 g sliced mango: 28 g carbs/3 g from fiber
- 1 medium pear: 28 g carbs/6 g from fiber

On the other hand, berries have more fiber and less sugar than most other fruits, so- even on a low carb diet- you can enjoy them in moderation (1/2 cup, or 50 grams).

Starchy Veggies

Most diets- even low carb ones- do allow you to have an unlimited consumption of low starch veggies. After all, most veggies are high fiber, which can help maximize weight loss and balance glucose levels. On the other hand, there are some veggies that are high starch that contain less fiber and more carbs, and therefore should be limited on low carb diets.

If you're trying to stick to a very low carb diet, it's best to avoid the following completely:

- 1 cup/175 g corn: 41 g carbs/5 g from fiber
- 1 medium potato: 37 g carbs/4 g from fiber
- 1 medium sweet potato/yam: 24 g carbs/4 g from fiber
- 1 cup/150 g cooked beets: 16 g carbs/4 g from fiber

Again, most low carb diets do allow you to have lots of low carb veggies.

Pasta

Pasta is versatile and cheap- so it's great for those who are on a budget. However, it's very high in carbs, so it's not ideal for those who are on a low carb diet. In fact, 1 cup/250 grams of pasta has 43 grams carbs- and only 3 of those are from fiber. Don't assume that whole wheat pasta is much better: one serving has 37 grams of carbs- and only 6 grams are from fiber.

Therefore, if you're on a low carb diet, spaghetti or other pasta isn't really the best idea unless you eat a smaller portion- which, truthfully, is not easy for most people. If you really can't give up your pasta, consider trying some shirataki noodles or spiralizing some veggies instead (zucchini makes great noodles).

Breakfast Cereal

We all know that the sugary breakfast cereals are full of carbs- but are you aware that even the so-called "healthy" options have high carb counts too? For example, 1 cup/90 grams of cooked oatmeal contains 32 grams carbs, only 4 from fiber.

Even steel cut oats, which are considered healthier, because they're not as processed as most other forms of oatmeal are not a great option: ½ cup/45 grams contains 29 grams carbs, 5 from fiber.

The whole grain cereals are even worse: a ½ cup/61 gram serving of granola contains 37 grams carbs, 7 from fiber. The same serving size of Grape Nuts contains 46 grams carbs, 5 from fiber.

Therefore, it's best to avoid (or at least minimize) breakfast cereals when you're on a low-carb diet because one serving could very easily throw you over the limit- before you even add the milk.

Beer

Even if you're on a low carb diet, you don't have to completely give up alcohol. You can still enjoy it in moderation. After all, hard liquor contains zero carbs and dry wines have very few. However, beer is actually full of carbs. In fact, one 12-oz/356 ml can contains 12 grams of carbs- and even light beers contain 6 grams per can.

Some experts caution that liquid carbs actually cause weight gain more than carbs from solid foods because they're not as filling and don't really satiate your appetite as much as food does. Therefore, if you still want to enjoy alcohol from time to time on your low carb diet, try spirits or dry wines.

Sweetened Yogurt

Yogurt is both versatile and tasty. While it's true that plain yogurt typically has a fairly low carb count, most people prefer to enjoy fruity, sweet non-fat/low-fat varieties. Unfortunately, these sweetened varieties contain high carb counts.

In fact, 1 cup/245 grams of sweetened, nonfat fruit yogurt typically has around 47 grams carbs, much higher than a serving of ice cream the same size. However, if you choose ½ cup/123 grams of plain Greek yogurt with ½ cup/50 grams of raspberries or blackberries will keep the carb count less than 10 grams.

Juice

When you commit to a low carb diet, juices are a terrible idea. While it's true that it provides you some nutrients, it's packed with quickly digesting carbs that cause a blood sugar spike. For example, a 12 oz/355 ml glass of apple juice contains 48 grams of carbs- more than soda, which contains 39 g. Additionally, a 12 oz/355 ml serving of grape juice contains 60 grams of carbs.

Finally, juice is liquid carbs, so your brain doesn't process it in the same way that it does solid carbs. When you drink juices, it can actually cause you to be hungrier and end up eating more later on during the day.

Low-Fat/Fat-Free Salad Dressings

Since salads are made up of non-starchy veggies, you can enjoy a plethora of salads when you're on a low carb diet. However, you should be aware that the low-fat/fat free salad dressings actually add more carbs than you might think. For example:

- 2 Tbsp/30 ml Fat-Free French Dressing: 10 grams carbs
- 2 Tbsp/30 ml Fat-Free Ranch Dressing: 11 grams carbs

The worst part is that even though the suggested serving size is 2 Tbsp/30 ml, most people actually use more than that- especially on a large salad. If you want to decrease your carb count, it's best to use a creamy, full-fat dressing instead. On the other hand, you might want to consider simply using olive oil and vinegar- which, according to experts, has been proven to improve the health of your heart and could potentially assist in weight loss.

Beans/Legumes

Beans/legumes are high in nutrition and have many benefits, including decreasing inflammation and your risk for heart disease- but they are high in carbs. Depending upon your carb limits, these could be included in your low carb diet.

Following are the carb counts for one serving of cooked beans/legumes:

- Lentils: 40 grams carbs/16 g from fiber
- Peas: 25 grams carbs/9 g from fiber
- Black beans: 41 grams carbs/15 g from fiber
- Pinto beans: 45 grams carbs/15 g from fiber
- Chickpeas: 45 grams carbs/12 g from fiber
- Kidney beans: 40 grams carbs/13 g from fiber

As you can see, beans/legumes are healthy- but are high in carbs. How-ever, you don't have to necessarily cut them out completely, you can con-sume small amounts, depending upon your personal carb limits.

Honey/Sugar (any kind)

You already know that foods containing white sugar, such as cakes, candy, and cookies are a "no-go" on a low carb diet. What you may not be aware of is that even natural forms of sugar can have as many- if not more- carbs than white sugar when you measure them in tablespoons. Following are the carbohydrate counts for 1 Tbsp of various types of sugar:

- White sugar: 12.6 g
- Maple syrup: 13 g
- Agave nectar: 16 g
- Honey: 17 g

Additionally, these don't really bring any other nutritional value to the table. When you are limiting your carbs, it's critical that you choose sources that are nutritious and high in fiber. In order to sweeten foods/drinks without increasing carb count, choose a healthy sweetener.

Chips/Crackers

When it comes to snack time, many people reach for chips and/or crackers. However, the carbs from these foods can add up quite quickly. An average serving size of tortilla chips is 10-15 chips/1 oz/28 grams and contains 18 grams carbs/1 gram from fiber. The carb counts in crackers varies depend-ing on the way they are processed. Still, even whole wheat crackers have about 19 grams of carbs- 3 from fiber- in a 1 oz/28 gram serving. Most people consume large amounts of these snack foods in a short amount of time- so if you're on a low carb diet, it's best if you just completely avoid them.

Milk

You know that milk "does a body good"- after all, it supplies your body with various nutrients, including: B vitamins, calcium, and potassium. However, the issue is the carb count-an 8 oz/240 ml serving contains 12-13 g carbs, whether it's whole milk, low-fat, or fat-free.

Of course, if you're only using 1-2 Tbsp/15-30 ml in your coffee one time a day, you can include milk in your low-carb diet- but cream/half-and-half are much better if you drink a lot of coffee since the carb count in these are much lower. If you like to drink milk or make lattes/smoothies, you might want to substitute almond or coconut milk.

Gluten-Free Baked Goods

In recent years, gluten-free diets have become quite popular- and are necessary for those who have celiac disease, a condition that causes the gut to be inflamed when gluten is consumed. Gluten is a protein that is found in products containing rye, barley, and wheat.

So, while gluten-free is a necessary option if you have this condition, it's not the best option if you're dieting- especially if you're on a low carb diet. This is because gluten-free products typically contain more carbs than the regular versions. In addition, the flour that is used in these products often contains grains/starches that result in a glucose spike.

Therefore, if you're on a low-carb diet, you really should choose whole foods. However, if you need baked goods, bake them at home with coconut or almond flour instead of reaching for those gluten-free products.

The bottom line is this: if you're on a low-carb diet, it's necessary to choose nutritious foods that are low in carbs. As you see, some foods must be eliminated, while you can enjoy many others- as long as you practice moderation. The choices that you make depend upon your personal carb limit.

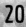

What am I Allowed to Eat?

After reading the section above, you may feel like switching to a low-carb lifestyle may not be for you because there are so many things you must avoid. However, don't feel like this! There are plenty of things that you can still enjoy. In this section, you will find a list of the foods that you can still enjoy on a low-carb diet.

Meat

You can eat any type of meat that you like on a low-carb diet: beef, poultry, pork, game, and lamb. Of course, you will want to remove the skin on the chicken and you might be better to choose meats that are organic or grass fed.

Fish/Seafood

You can eat any type of seafood on a low-carb diet as well: herring, sardines, salmon, and mackerel are all great option. Additionally, since they're high in omega-3 fatty acids, they may offer some other health benefits as well. However, you will want to avoid breading them, as that will add carbs.

Eggs

If possible, you'll want to try to get organic eggs- but you can enjoy eggs cooked in any way: omelets, fried, boiled, and scrambled.

Natural Fats/High-Fat Sauces

You already know that using butter or cream when you cook makes food taste better, right? Plus, cooking this way can make you feel more satiated. Consider adding a Hollandaise or Bearnaise sauce to your meals. If you're using one that is pre-made, make sure to read the label and check for veggie oils and starches. If possible, you'll want to make it for yourself. Other good options include olive oil and coconut oil, as they are healthy fats.

Veggies

The following veggies have low carb counts, so you can enjoy them on an

y of the low-carb diet/lifestyles: asparagus, avocado, bok choy, broccoli, Brussels sprouts, cabbage, cauliflower, collards, cucumber, eggplant, kale, lettuce, mushrooms, olives, onion, peppers, spinach, tomatoes, zucchini, and other leafy greens. Of course, if you're following the keto diet, you must consume no more than 20 g carbs/day, you may want to pay attention to your portions of certain types of veggies such as Brussels sprouts and bell peppers.

Dairy

You'll want to be careful with whole, skim, and low fat milk because they contain high amounts of milk sugar. However, you can enjoy full fat options of sour cream, real butter, Greek/Turkish yogurt, cheese, and cream. All of these will keep you full and satisfied. The biggest thing to remember with dairy is to avoid low-fat, sugary, and flavored products.

Nuts

If you're craving a snack, reach for nuts instead of candy, chips, or popcorn

Berries

These are a great option- in moderation- if you are craving something sweet and you don't need to watch your carbs too closely. They're really great with whipped cream.

Drinks

It's important to stay hydrated at all times, whether you're on a low carb diet or not. However, it becomes a bit more challenging when you are on a low carb diet.

- Water is always the best choice in all situations. You can reach for sparkling or flavored water if you wish, but you'll want to double check the labels for added sugars, as well as the carb count.

- Coffee/Tea is an acceptable option but needs to be plain or with a small amount of milk/cream. If you drink coffee throughout the day, you'll want to avoid adding a lot of milk/cream when you're not hungry. You can use butter and coconut oil or full-fat cream when you're hungry.

Celebrations/Special Events

What if you're celebrating or you've been invited out with friends? Don't worry too much about it- you don't have to completely go off the rails with your diet. Sure, it's true that a lot of celebrating can slow your progress if you're trying to lose weight- just get back to your diet as soon as you can and you'll continue to lose weight.

- Alcohol: you can enjoy alcohol such as sparkling wine, champagne, gin, dry wine, whisky, vodka, and brandy in moderation.
- Chocolate: chocolate is not off limits on a low carb diet- but needs to be dark chocolate, more than 70% cocoa, and only in small amounts.
- Dark chocolate: small amounts of 70% or higher cocoa

How Many Carbs Should I Consume Each Day?

Before we start to explore the low-carb lifestyle, you'll want to take the time to determine your personal daily carb limit so that you can know how much you can comfortably cut back to. When you ask how many carbs you should be consuming, you'll probably get an answer like this: It depends. While this isn't really an exciting answer, it's the best one because after all, the carbs that you need is determined by your body's makeup, your activity level, and whether or not you have any underlying medical issues. In addition, your needs may fluctuate, depending on were you are in your cycle or the time of year.

Individuals with SAD, or seasonal affective disorder, are likely to reach for carb-rich foods during the darker months, due to the fact that their serotonin dips. Carb consumption helps with serotonin production, which explains why we crave carbs on emotionally draining days.

According to the 2015-2020 Dietary Guidelines, 45-65% of our daily calories should be from carbs. This means that on the typical 2,000 calorie diet, we should be consuming 225-325 grams. The minimum recommended amount of carbs is 130 grams, which is about eight to nine 15-gram servings daily.

If you're interested in starting a low-carb diet and you want to track your macronutrients, you can make changes to your carb:protein:fat ratio until you find the balance that allows you to meet your goals but also feels sustainable. Keep in mind that if you're not consuming enough carbs, you will typically feel mentally drained and sluggish. Additionally, you may have a hard time keeping yourself together emotionally. On the other hand, if you consume too many carbs, you don't stay full for very long because your body is burning through your meals/snacks quickly. This is the cause of the "blood sugar roller coaster", which could potentially result in insulin resistance and prediabetes.

It's best to include carbs in every meal. The way that you incorporate them is entirely up to you. However, when you spread your carbs out through the day, you keep your glucose levels stable, which balances your mood and energy levels.

How to Get Started on a Low Carb Eating Plan

So far, we have explored what carbs are, how they react in our body, and what low carb really means. In this section, we will take a look at the steps you'll need to follow in order to get started on a low carb diet/lifestyle.

As you can see, low carb diets are conducive to weight loss. However, when it comes right down to it, it's a bit daunting to do. If you are like most, it is going to require some drastic changes and significant commitment. While there's tons of information out there, you need some practical tips that you can easily incorporate into your life.

First of all, you must start by slowly reducing your consumption of simple carbs and increasing your consumption of complex carbs. Once you've done that, you can start making some low-carb swaps. Additionally, keep in mind that you can make smarter meal choices to keep you fuller longer. If you plan on sticking with this low carb eating plan for the long haul, you'll want to do some research and settle on a specific diet plan so that you can have access to helpful tools and a community of others for support.

Reduce Carb Consumption

When it comes to reducing your carb consumption, the very first thing you must do is cut out all simple carbohydrates and refined sugars. Of course, you should not cut them out all at once, that would be too much. In order to make the process more bearable, it's best to cut them out one at a time. Start by replacing sugary drinks/sodas with sugar-free drinks and water. Some popular sources of simple carbs/refined sugars include: candy, white bread, sodas/sugary drinks, cookies/cakes/baked goods, white rice, pasta, and potatoes.

As you transition away from these simple carbohydrates and refined sugars, switch to whole grains. Before you go all in with the low-carb way of life, consider replacing some of your simple carbs with whole grain options. Once again, start out slowly, replacing one serving of your typical carbohydrate with a whole grain option every day for about one week. After a week or so, you'll find that you're not eating nearly as many simple carbs and choosing more complex carbs. This reduces your overall carb consumption, and (bonus!) you'll feel full and satisfied longer. Here are a few complex carb options to keep in mind: steel-cut oatmeal, brown rice, high-fiber/low-sugar cereal, and whole wheat pastas and breads.

As stated previously, white potatoes are considered a simple carb. Therefore, as you transition into your new low-carb lifestyle, you'll want to swap them for sweet potatoes/root veggies. You can bake/use sweet potatoes and other root veggies just as you would white potatoes. Some great options include the following: baked sweet potatoes/yams, mashed turnips/rutabaga, roasted beets/carrots/kohlrabi, and celery root/daikon radish fries.

When you're ready to transition into your new low carb lifestyle/diet, it's best to try simple swaps to decrease your carb consumption. Here are a few simple swaps you can make that won't leave you feeling deprived of your favorite foods:

- Instead of white rice, choose cauliflower rice. Take your food processor/box grater and shred a head of cauliflower into rice-like chunks. You can then cook it by microwaving for 3 to 4 minutes and then use it for any recipe that calls for rice.

- Instead of pasta noodles, use spaghetti squash or zucchini noodles. You can use a vegetable peeler/mandoline slicer to make zucchini noodles or bake spaghetti squash, scoop out seeds and scape out strands. Then, top with your favorite pasta sauce and enjoy.

- Instead of snacking on potato chips, munch on raw veggies or nuts instead. There are times when you need something crunchy to snack on- but instead of wasting those calories on potato chips, choose something healthy, such as a handful of nuts or fresh carrots or celery.

- Instead of reaching for candy or baked goods, choose berries. They are low in carbs, but high in other nutrients. Plus, they're as sweet- if not sweeter- than candy. If you have a craving for something sweet, grab a handful of raspberries, strawberries, or blueberries.

Stay Full & Satisfied

When you switch to a new way of eating, it can be difficult to stay full and satisfied. After all, you're used to eating those simple carbs- all day long. However, when you cut back on carbs, you have to make more of an effort to make good food choices. Even though you won't be eating as much, these tips will ensure you stay full and satisfied.

Proteins should be the primary focus of your meals- but that can lead to cholesterol issues, right? Choose lean proteins that have lower fat content such as the following: canned tuna in water, tofu, ground turkey, egg whites, skinless chicken, cottage cheese (low-fat), or lean ground beef.

While you do have to cut back on starchy veggies on low-carb diets, most of them will allow you to eat an unlimited amount of non-starchy veggies, which help keep you full. Here are a few options to choose from: broccoli, cabbage, cauliflower, cucumbers, eggplant, peppers, spinach, and zucchini.

For many people, snacking is a major problem when switching to a low carb diet- but you can keep yourself full and satisfied by stocking your fridge/pantry with plenty of low carb snack options. Here are a few great options: beef jerky, plain Greek yogurt, fresh veggies (such as broccoli, celery, peppers, etc), boiled eggs, or raw almonds.

Making the effort to stay hydrated on a low carb diet will also do wonders for helping you feel full and satisfied- plus, it will help you avoid dehydration. The best option is to drink water and unsweetened drinks because when you drink sugar-free sodas/artificially sweetened drinks, it can actually trigger your sweet tooth, which is not something you want. Here are a few great beverage options: coffee, unsweetened tea, or sparkling water.

Choose a Diet You Can Stick With Long-Term

Since the low carb movement has gained so much popularity, there are several options to choose from when it comes to diets. However, you want to do some research and find one that works for you for the long term. You don't want to bounce around from diet to diet- you want something that you can make work for you. Here is a little bit of information on some of the more popular ones:

Atkins

If you want a classic low-carb diet, Atkins is an excellent choice. It has been around for a few years and many people have been successful on it, which means it's a great place to start your low-carb journey. According to Atkins experts, you can lose around 15 pounds (6.8 kg) within the first two weeks you're on it. Therefore, if you need to quickly shed a lot of weight, this is a great plan.

Getting Started with Atkins

For the first two weeks, you will have to cut down to 20 g carbs/day. In addition, you'll have to completely eliminate refined sugars/simple carbs. Other things you'll have to cut out the first two weeks are: starchy veggies such as corn, potatoes, and broccoli; nuts and whole grains. As you continue following the Atkins plan, you'll add these in slowly.

Atkins requires that you have some form of protein with every meal. You can keep things interesting by trying something new every few nights. Take some time to experiment with turkey, fish, chicken, and even tofu.

Atkins is great for those who struggle with health conditions such as high blood pressure, cardiovascular disease, metabolic syndrome, or diabetes.

There are some claims that Atkins has improved these conditions- and some have even claimed that Atkins reversed their condition.

South Beach Diet

If your primary goal for going low carb is to develop healthy eating habits, you might want to consider the South Beach Diet. A cardiologist developed the South Beach Diet and it will not only help with weight loss, but also encourages healthy eating habits. Another good thing about the South Beach Diet is that it doesn't restrict carbs as much as some of the other diet plans, so many people find that it's much easier to stick to in the long run.

Getting Started with South Beach Diet

1. **Phase 1:** Cut out all carbs
2. **Phase 2:** Begin to slowly re-introduce healthy carbs into your diet (1-2 servings/day)
3. **Phase 3:** Add carbs back into your diet- practicing the art of moderation

The South Beach Diet does guide you to choose carbs with a low glycemic index, which will help moderate your hunger and blood sugar. Also, this diet encourages you to choose monosaturated fats, which are heart-healthy. Finally, the South Beach Diet promotes fruit (in moderation), veggies, and lean proteins.

Ketogenic Diet

Lately, the ketogenic diet is extremely popular, and is great for those who want a meal plan that is both satisfying and high in fat. The focus of this plan is to increase your daily calories to the following: 75% fat, 5% carbs, and 20% protein, which encourages your body to use up your fat stores, leading to quick weight loss.

According to the experts, the ketogenic diet has been proven to benefit those who have been diagnosed with epilepsy- but it may also help with the prevention of dementia, Alzheimer's, and stroke and help people heal from traumatic brain injury. However, there are potential side effects such as moodiness, brain fog, and fatigue as you change your eating habits.

Dukan Diet

If you need a structured plan to get you started in your new low-carb life-style, try the Dukan diet. It's one of the most structured plans you'll find. For the first ten days of this diet plan, you're only allowed to eat oat bran, lean protein, and drink water. After ten days, you can add non-starchy veggies, hard cheese, one serving of fruit, and a serving of whole grains. According to the experts, you may lose 10 pounds/4.5 kg in the first two weeks, and about 2 to 4 pounds/0.91 to 1.8 kg after that.

Of course, one of the issues with the Dukan diet is the restrictions. You are at risk for some nutritional deficiencies.

Paleo Diet

Another popular option is the Paleo diet, which is a great option if you want to put emphasis on whole foods. On this diet, you must cut out all pro-cessed foods, dairy, potatoes, and grains. You can eat your fill of fruits, roots, veggies, nuts, and meat- which will help you stay full and satisfied. This plan is healthy because of the emphasis on whole foods.

Paleo diet experts believe that many of today's health issues are due to our diet, which include lots of grains and dairy.

Stay Healthy & Motivated

The hardest part of any lifestyle change is staying motivated. However, it can be done- just keep the following in mind:

If you have a diagnosed medical condition, be sure to speak with your physician before making any changes to your diet. They will be able to advise you on whether a low carb diet is good for your situation. Additionally, they can help you choose the right one.

For example, if you have been diagnosed with diabetes, it's probably best if you swap out healthy carbs such as whole grains and fruits, instead of eliminating all carbs. If you have high cholesterol, it's not good to choose foods high in saturated fats and cholesterol. Your physician suggest that you choose lean proteins: egg whites, skinless poultry, and low-fat cottage cheese.

One great way to keep up with your carbs, is to use a tracking app. Of course, you will have to be committed to logging everything you eat. This will help you keep track of the carbs/macros you're consuming. Some apps even have a function where you can store recipes, make grocery lists, and even plan meals.

On the other hand, some people prefer to write things down- and there's nothing wrong with that. Simply grab a journal/notebook and write down everything each day. You can use the food labels to find the nutrition information. If there's not a food label, take the time to look up the calories, carbs, protein, and fat in a guidebook or online.

One way to keep yourself on track is to take the time to prep meals ahead of time. Simply set aside a few hours one day to find a few recipes and put together some (if not all) of your meals for the week. This way, you're less likely to come home after a long day at work and choose unhealthy take out over a healthier at home option. Here are a few tips for prepping your meals ahead of time:

- Prep ingredients. Take time to chop up any veggies that you need for your meals during the week. Then, measure them out and place them in separate containers for cooking.
- Cook proteins. If possible, go ahead and cook your proteins so that you just need to heat them up when you're ready. Bake salmon, grill chicken, boil eggs, and prepare other protein as desired.
- Portion meals. Take the time to portion your meals into single serving containers so that you can grab and go. An example would be 4 oz/35 g grilled chicken (skinless), 1 c/91 g steamed broccoli, and 1 c/150 g baked zucchini.

Many people find their motivation to keep going by connecting with a community of others who are following the same diet. This will give you somewhere to turn when you have questions or concerns about starting or sticking to the diet. They can give you tips/advice- and you can help them as well. You can find communities online or in your local area. However, when you join, don't just sit idle- get involved!

When you join, introduce yourself and let them know that you're just getting started and you could use some help. When you struggle, don't hesitate to reach out to others for some support. For example, if you're struggling with sweet cravings, ask others what they've done to combat those cravings. Chances are, they've been there (or maybe still are) and can offer you some advice.

LOW CARB RECIPES

LOW CARB BREAKFAST RECIPES

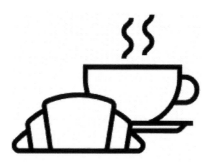

GOAT CHEESE & HERB OMELET

Time: 10 mins | Serves 1

Nutrition Information: Calories: 523/Calories from fat: 387 | Fat: 24 g | Cholesterol: 709 mg | Protein: 31 g | Carbs: 3 g

What You'll Need:

- 3 eggs
- 1 Tbsp butter, unsalted
- 2 oz fresh goat cheese
- 1 Tbsp chopped herbs such as basil, cilantro, or parsley
- Salt & black pepper (to taste)

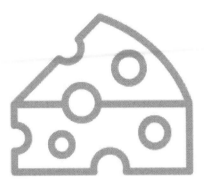

What You'll Do:

1. In a bowl, whisk together eggs, salt, pepper, and herbs.
2. In skillet, melt butter.
3. Once hot, add eggs and cook about 3-4 mins- until set.
4. Crumble goat cheese and fold over.
5. Cook until cheese is melty- about 1 min.

FRITTATA WITH SPINACH & GOAT CHEESE

Nutrition Information: Calories: 399 | Fat: 31 g | Cholesterol: 551 mg | Protein: 23 g | Carbohydrates: 9 g

What You'll Need:

♦   3 Tbsps olive oil

♦   ½ medium-size onion, sliced thin

♦   5 oz (6 cups) baby spinach

♦   10 large eggs

♦   4 oz (1 cup) goat cheese crumbles

♦   1 Tbsp white wine vinegar

♦   5 oz (6 cups) mixed greens

♦   Kosher salt/black pepper (to taste)

♦   Country bread

What You'll Do:

1.   Preheat oven to 400□F/204□C.

2.   In medium nonstick, ovenproof skillet, heat 1 Tbsp olive oil.

3.   Place onion, along with salt & pepper in skillet and saute until golden- about 3-4 mins.

4.   Add baby spinach and cook until wilted, 1-2 mins.

5.   Add eggs and sprinkle goat cheese on top. Cook until eggs begin to set around edges, 1-2 mins.

6.   Place in oven and bake until set, about 10-12 mins.

7.   In a large bowl, whisk together remaining 2 Tbsp oil, salt & pepper, and vinegar.

8.   Add mixed greens, tossing to combine. Serve with country bread and frittata.

FRIED EGG SANDWICH

Total Time: 21 mins | Servings: 1

Nutrition Information: Calories: 477 | Fat: 36 g | Carbs: 1 g | Protein: 34 g | Cholesterol: 450 mg

What You'll Need:

♦ Nonstick cooking spray

♦ 3 slices bacon

♦ Salt & black pepper, to taste

♦ 2 eggs

♦ 1/3 c shredded cheddar cheese

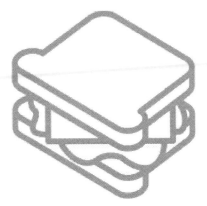

What You'll Do:

1. In skillet, brown bacon on medium high heat- about 10 mins.

2. Drain grease onto paper towels. Crumble, set aside.

3. In separate skillet, cook eggs until whites are set and firm- approximately 3-4 mins.

4. Flip and continue cooking.

5. Sprinkle bacon & cheese over one egg.

6. Continue cooking until eggs reach desired doneness and cheese is melty.

7. Place second egg on top and move to serving dish.

SPINACH QUICHE (NO CRUST)

Total Time: 50 mins | Servings: 6

Nutrition Information: Calories: 309 | Fat: 23 g | Carbs: 4 g | Protein: 20 g | Cholesterol: 209 mg

What You'll Need:

- 1 Tbsp vegetable oil
- 5 eggs
- 1 onion, chopped
- Salt & black pepper, as desired
- 3 c shredded muenster cheese
- 10-oz bag frozen (thawed/drained) spinach, chopped

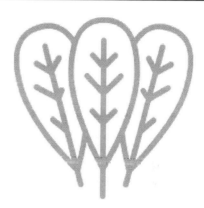

What You'll Do:

1. Preheat oven to 350□F/175□C.
2. Lightly grease 9-inch pie pan.
3. Place oil in skillet and heat on med-high heat. Add onions, cook until soft.
4. Add spinach and cook until excess moisture is evaporated.
5. In separate bowl, combine salt, pepper, eggs, and cheese.
6. Stir in spinach and place mixture in pie pan.
7. Place in oven and bake about 30 mins, or until eggs have set.
8. Cool for 10 mins before serving.

EGG & CHEESE BOATS

Total Time: 43 mins | Servings: 2

Nutrition Information: Calories: 578 | Fat: 44 g | Carbs: 7 g | Protein: 38 g | Cholesterol: 482 mg

What You'll Need:

- 4 eggs
- 2 oval sandwich rolls
- 3 Tbsp whole milk
- 1 (4-oz) can chopped green chili peppers
- 1 c shredded cheddar cheese
- ½ c pepper Jack cheese, shredded
- ½ tsp smoked paprika
- ¼ tsp salt

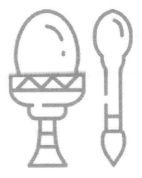

What You'll Do:

1. Preheat oven to 350F/175C.
2. Use parchment paper to line baking sheet.
3. Cut a v-shape in each roll, but leave the ends together.
4. Lift out the wedge and hollow out rolls to make bread bowls.
5. Take care that you don't cut through the bottom or sides of the rolls.
6. Place rolls on baking sheet.
7. Crack eggs and pour milk into separate bowl and whisk until blended.
8. Stir in chili peppers, cheeses, salt, and paprika.
9. Slowly pour into prepared rolls, using a spoon to spread evenly.
10. Bake for 20 mins or until set and cheese is browned.
11. Allow to cool for 3 mins before serving.

SAUSAGE CASSEROLE

Total Time: 1 h 45 mins | Servings: 12

Nutrition Information: Calories: 355 | Fat: 26 g | Carbs: 8 g | Protein: 21 g | Cholesterol: 188 mg

What You'll Need:

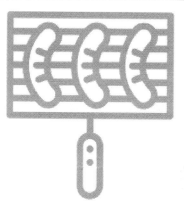

- 1 lb breakfast sausage, sage flavored
- 3 c shredded potatoes,
- ¼ c melted butter
- 12 oz shredded cheddar cheese
- ½ c shredded onion
- 1 (16-oz) container cottage cheese, small curd
- 6 jumbo eggs

What You'll Do:

1. Preheat oven to 375□F/190□C.
2. Grease 9x13 baking dish.
3. Brown sausage in skillet over med-high heat until evenly browned. Drain. Set aside.
4. In baking dish, stir butter and potatoes together. Line sides and bottom with potatoes.
5. Mix onion, eggs, sausage, cheese, and cottage cheese in separate bowl and pour over potatoes.
6. Bake for about 1 hour.
7. Allow to rest for 5 mins before cutting and serving.

OVEN SCRAMBLED EGGS

Total Time: 35 mins | Servings: 12

Nutrition Information: Calories: 236 | Fat: 18 g | Carbs: 3 g | Protein: 14 g | Cholesterol: 396 mg

What You'll Need:

- ♦ ½ c melted butter/margarine
- ♦ 24 eggs
- ♦ ¼ tsp salt
- ♦ ½ c milk

What You'll Do:

1. Preheat oven to 350°F/175°C.
2. Pour melted butter into baking dish.
3. In separate bowl, whisk eggs and salt until blended. Slowly blend in milk.
4. Pour into baking dish and place in oven, uncovered for 10 mins.
5. After 10 mins, stir and bake for 10-15 additional mins, or until eggs are set.

OVEN-BAKED DENVER OMELET

Total Time: 45 mins | Servings: 4

Nutrition Information: Calories: 345 | Fat: 26 g | Carbs: 3 g | Protein: 22 g | Cholesterol: 381 mg

What You'll Need:

♦ 2 Tbsp butter

♦ ½ each green bell pepper & onion, chopped

♦ 1 c chopped cooked ham

♦ 8 eggs

♦ ¼ c milk

♦ ½ c cheddar cheese, shredded

♦ Salt & black pepper, to taste

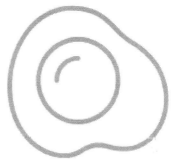

What You'll Do:

1. Preheat oven to 400□F/200□C.

2. Grease 10-in round baking dish.

3. Over medium heat, melt butter in skillet.

4. Cook bell pepper and onion about 5 mins.

5. Add ham and continue to cook until heated through, about 5 more mins.

6. In separate bowl, combine milk and eggs.

7. Add ham & cheese mixture and season as desired.

8. Pour into prepared baking dish.

9. Bake until eggs are puffy & brown, about 25 mins. Serve warm.

HAM, CHEESE, & HASHBROWN CASSEROLE

Total Time: 1 hr 15 mins | Servings: 12

Nutrition Information: Calories: 415 | Fat: 27 g | Carbs: 30 g | Protein: 14 g | Cholesterol: 53 mg

What You'll Need:

♦ 1 (32-oz) package frozen hash browns

♦ 8 ounce cooked ham, diced

♦ 2 c shredded sharp cheddar cheese

♦ 1 ½ c grated paremesan

♦ 2 (10.75 oz) cans cream of potato soup

♦ 16-oz sour cream

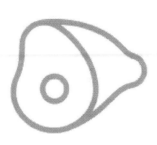

What You'll Do:

1. Preheat oven to 375□F/190□C.

2. Lightly grease 9x13 casserole dish.

3. In separate bowl, mix cheddar cheese, soup, hash browns, sour cream, and ham.

4. Spread mixture into casserole dish and sprinkle parmesan on top.

5. Bake until bubbly and light brown- about 1 hour.

FRENCH TOAST

Total Time: 30 mins | Servings: 12

Nutrition Information: Calories: 123 | Fat: 2 g | Carbs: 18 | Protein: 5 g | Cholesterol: 48 mg

What You'll Need:

♦ ¼ c flour, all purpose

♦ 1 c milk

♦ 1 pinch salt

♦ 3 eggs

♦ ½ tsp cinnamon

♦ 1 tsp vanilla extract

♦ 1 Tbsp white sugar

♦ 12 slices bread

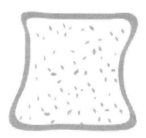

What You'll Do:

1. Put flour into large mixing bowl and slowly add milk.

2. Then add eggs, salt, vanilla extract, cinnamon, and sugar until mixture is smooth.

3. Place pan/griddle on medium heat.

4. Soak bread in mixture until saturated.

5. Cook until golden brown.

LOW CARB LUNCH RECIPES

CHIPPED BEEF ON TOAST

Total Time: 20 mins | Servings: 4

Nutrition Information: Calories: 197 | Fat: 9 g | Carbs: 9 g | Protein: 21 g | Cholesterol: 67 mg

What You'll Need:

♦ 2 Tbsp butter

♦ 2 Tbsp flour, all-purpose

♦ ½ c milk, warm

♦ 1 (8-oz) jar dried beef

♦ 1 pinch cayenne pepper

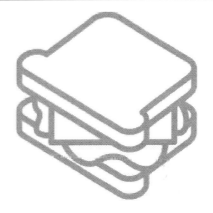

What You'll Do:

1. On low heat, melt butter in medium-size saucepan.

2. Whisk in flour to create roux.

3. Slowly add milk and increase to med-high heat. Continue to cook until mixture has thickened and bring to a boil.

4. Then, stir in cayenne and beef and heat through. Serve on toast.

LOW CARB BURGER

Total Time: 20 mins | Servings: 6

Nutrition Information: Calories: 323 | Fat: 17 g | Carbs: 10 g | Protein: 30 g | Cholesterol: 122 mg

What You'll Need:

- 2 lbs ground beef, extra lean
- 1 (1 Oz) package onion soup mix
- 1 egg
- 2 tsp each Worcestershire sauce and hot sauce
- ¼ tsp black pepper
- ¾ c rolled oats

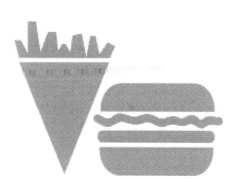

What You'll Do:

1. Preheat outdoor grill and lightly oil grate.
2. In small bowl, lightly beat egg.
3. In a separate large bowl, combine beef, egg, oats, onion soup mix, and hot sauce.
4. Create 6 patties from mixture.
5. Place patties on grill and grill on med-high heat for 10-20 mins, until they reach desired doneness.

BEEF DIP SANDWICH

Total Time: 6 h 10 mins | Servings: 10

Nutrition Information: Calories: 290 | Fat: 20 g |Carbs: 2 g (more if eaten on bread) | Protein: 23 g | Cholesterol: 82 mg

What You'll Need:

♦ 4 lbs beef chuck roast

♦ 1 Tbsp garlic, minced

♦ 1 Tbsp dried rosemary

♦ 3 bay leaves

♦ 1 c soy sauce

♦ 6 c water

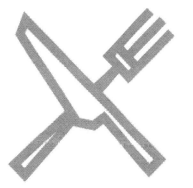

What You'll Do:

1. Season roast with garlic and rosemary.

2. Place roast and bay leaves in slow cooker and pour water and soy sauce in.

3. Cook on low for 6-10 hours.

4. Keep in mind, with this roast, the longer it cooks, the better it is.

5. When roast is done, remove from slow cooker and shred. Enjoy with or without bread.

GARLIC SALMON

Total Time: 40 mins | Servings: 6

Nutrition Information: Calories: 169 | Fat: 7 g | Carbs: 2 g | Protein: 24 g | Cholesterol: 50 mg

What You'll Need:

- ♦ 1 ½ lbs salmon filet
- ♦ Salt & black pepper (to taste)
- ♦ 3 cloves garlic, minced
- ♦ 1 sprig fresh dill
- ♦ 5 sprigs fresh dill weed
- ♦ 5 slices lemon
- ♦ 2 green onions, chopped

What You'll Do:

1. Preheat oven to 450▢F/230▢C and spray 2 large pieces of foil with cooking spray.
2. Place salmon on top of one piece of foil.
3. Sprinkle with garlic, chopped dill, salt, and pepper.
4. Arrange lemon on top and place one sprig of dill weed on top of each lemon.
5. Sprinkle with chopped green onion.
6. Cover with second piece of foil and pinch together to seal.
7. Place in large baking dish.
8. Bake for 20-25 mins, until flaky.

BACON & FETA STUFFED CHICKEN BREASTS

Total Time: 45 mins | Servings: 4

Nutrition Information: Calories: 451 | Fat: 35 g | Carbs: 3 g | Protein: 32 g | Cholesterol: 93 mg

What You'll Need:

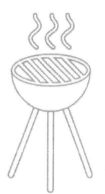

- 8 Tbsp olive oil
- 4 chicken breasts (boneless/skinless)
- 2 tsp lemon juice
- 1 Tbsp oregano
- 4 cloves garlic, crushed
- Salt & black pepper (as desired)
- 4 slices each bacon (fried/drained) and feta cheese

What You'll Do:

1. Preheat oven to 350□F/175□C.
2. In small bowl, mix together salt, pepper, lemon juice, oil, oregano, and garlic.
3. Slice chicken breasts halfway through to make an opening to place bacon and feta into.
4. Line 9x13 inch baking dish with foil and place chicken in dish.
5. Stuff each one with 1 slice each bacon and feta.
6. Secure open sides with toothpicks.
7. Drizzle with lemon juice mixture and place in oven.
8. Bake uncovered for about 30 mins.

TURKEY BURGERS WITH FETA CHEESE

Total Time: 20 mins | Servings: 4

Nutrition Information: Calories: 318 | Fat: 22 g | Carbs: 4 g | Protein: 26 g | Cholesterol: 123 mg

What You'll Need:

- 1 lb ground turkey
- 1 c feta cheese, crumbled
- ½ c kalamata olives, pitted & sliced
- 2 tsp oregano
- Black pepper (to taste)

What You'll Do:

1. Preheat grill to med-high and lightly oil grate.
2. In large bowl, mix together ground turkey, black pepper, oregano, feta cheese, and olives.
3. Form 4 patties from mixture.
4. Place patties on grill and cook for 10-12 mins, flipping over halfway through cook time.

HAM & CHEESE ROLLS

Total Time: 35 mins | Servings: 24

Nutrition Information: Calories: 145 | Fat: 9 g | Carbs: 10 g | Protein: 6 g | Cholesterol: 18 mg

What You'll Need:

- 2 Tbsp minced onion
- 1 Tbsp mustard
- 2 Tbsp poppy seeds
- ½ c melted margarine
- 24 dinner rolls
- ½ lb ham, chopped
- ½ lb Swiss cheese, thinly sliced

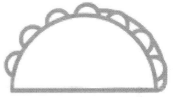

What You'll Do:

1. Preheat oven to 325☐F/165☐C.
2. In small bowl, mix together margarine, mustard, onion flakes, and poppy seeds.
3. Split each dinner roll and place ham and cheese inside to make a sandwich.
4. Arrange rolls on baking sheet and dribble melted margarine on top.
5. Bake until cheese is melty- about 20 mins.

BBQ BACON SHRIMP

Total Time: 45 mins | Servings: 3

Nutrition Information: Calories: 160 | Fat: 11 g | Carbs: 0.3 g | Protein: 15 g | Cholesterol: 83 mg

What You'll Need:

- 16 large shrimp, peeled/deveined
- 8 slices bacon
- BBQ seasoning

What You'll Do:

1. Preheat oven to 450☐F/230☐C.
2. Wrap shrimp with ½ slice bacon, secure with toothpick.

   Note: make sure to use large shrimp, as the cook time on the shrimp and bacon is similar. If you use medium-size shrimp, you'll want to precook your bacon, as overcooked shrimp are rubbery/tough.

3. Line pan with foil and place baking rack in pan.
4. Put shrimp on rack and sprinkle with BBQ seasoning.
5. Flip shrimp and sprinkle other side.
6. Let sit for about 15 mins so that seasonings can soak in.
7. Bacon will turn opaque, instead of being creamy white.
8. Bake in oven until bacon is crisp & shrimp tender, about 10-15 mins.

GRILLED MUSHROOMS

Total Time: 35 mins | Servings: 4

Nutrition Information: Calories: 156 | Fat: 14 g | Carbs: 7 g | Protein: 3 g | Cholesterol: 0 mg

What You'll Need:

- ½ c red bell pepper, finely chopped
- 1 garlic clove, minced
- ¼ c olive oil
- ¼ tsp onion powder
- Salt & black pepper, as desired
- 4 portobello mushroom caps

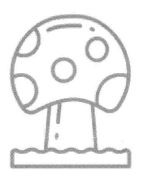

What You'll Do:

1. Preheat grill to medium and lightly oil grate.
2. In large bowl, combine black pepper, salt, garlic, red bell pepper, onion powder, and oil.
3. Spread on grill side of mushroom caps.
4. Place mushrooms to the side (over indirect heat) and cover.
5. Cook for 15-20 mins.

GRILLED TANDOORI CHICKEN

Total Time: 8 h 55 mins | Servings: 8

Nutrition Information: Calories: 349 | Fat: 21 g | Carbs: 5 g | Protein: 34 g | Cholesterol: 120 mg

What You'll Need:

- 12-oz plain yogurt
- Salt and black pepper, as desired
- ⅛ tsp ground cloves
- 2 Tbsp ginger, fresh grated
- 3 cloves garlic, finely minced
- 4 tsp paprika
- 2 tsp each cinnamon, coriander, and cumin
- 16 chicken thighs
- Olive oil spray

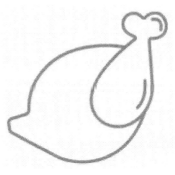

What You'll Do:

1. In medium bowl, combine ginger, salt, cloves, pepper, and yogurt.
2. Add coriander, cinnamon, garlic, cumin, and paprika and set aside.
3. Under cold water, carefully rinse chicken and then pat dry with paper towels and place in large zip-top bag.
4. Pour yogurt mixture over chicken and seal, making sure to press all air out of bag.
5. Turn over several times to distribute marinated evenly.
6. Place in bowl and refrigerate for 8 hours, turning occasionally.
7. Preheat grill to medium.
8. Remove chicken from bag and wipe off excess marinade.
9. Spray chicken with olive oil spray.
10. Place chicken on grill over direct heat and cook for 2 mins. Then, flip and cook 2 more mins. Move chicken to indirect heat and cook for 35-40 mins, until it reaches an internal temp of 180⸋F.

MEATBALLS W/ SWEET & SOUR SAUCE

Total Time: 1 h 50 mins | Servings: 12

Nutrition Information: Calories: 152 | Fat: 6 g | Carbs: 17 g | Protein: 8 g | Cholesterol: 38 mg

What You'll Need:

- 12-oz can/bottle chili sauce
- 2 tsp lemon juice
- 9-oz grape jelly
- 1 lb ground beef
- 1 egg (beaten)
- 1 large onion, grated
- Salt, as desired

What You'll Do:

1. Whisk together grape jelly, lemon juice, and chili sauce.
2. Pour into slow cooker and simmer until warm.
3. Combine ground beef, salt, egg, and onion.
4. Form meatballs from mixture and add to sauce. Simmer for 1 ½ hours.

HERBY LEMON CHICKEN

Total Time: 25 mins | Servings: 2

Nutrition Information: Calories: 212 | Fat: 9 g | Carbs: 8 g | Protein: 29 g | Cholesterol: 68 mg

What You'll Need:

- ♦ 2 chicken breast halves (boneless/skinless)
- ♦ Salt & black pepper, as desired
- ♦ 1 whole lemon
- ♦ 1 Tbsp olive oil
- ♦ 1 pinch oregano
- ♦ 2 sprigs parsley (garnish)

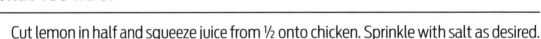

What You'll Do:

1. Cut lemon in half and squeeze juice from ½ onto chicken. Sprinkle with salt as desired.
2. Set aside while you heat oil in small skillet over med-low heat.
3. Once oil is heated, place chicken in skillet.
4. As you sauté, add juice from ½ lemon, oregano, and pepper to taste.
5. Sauté until juices run clear- about 5-10 mins on each side.

GYRO BURGER

Total Time: 25 mins | Servings: 4

Nutrition Information: Calories: 338 | Fat: 25 g | Carbs: 6 g | Protein: 20 g | Cholesterol: 84 mg

What You'll Need:

- ½ lb each lean ground beef and lamb
- ½ onion, grated
- 2 cloves garlic, pressed
- 1 slice toast, crumbled
- ½ tsp each dried savory, allspice, coriander, salt, and pepper
- 1 dash cumin

What You'll Do:

1. Preheat grill to med-high and lightly oil grate.
2. In large bowl, combine bread crumbs, lamb, beef, onion, and garlic.
3. Add cumin, savory, salt, allspice, pepper, and coriander.
4. Knead until mixture is well blended and shape into 4 thin patties.
5. Cook for about 5-7 mins on each side.

LOW CARB DINNER RECIPES

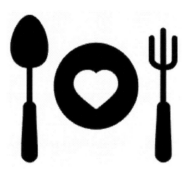

LASAGNA STUFFED PEPPERS

Total Time: 1 h 30 mins | Servings: 12

Nutrition Facts: Calories: 232 | Fat: 13 g | Carbs: 10 g | Protein: 18 g | Cholesterol: 49 mg

What You'll Need:

- 1 lb ground beef
- 3 8-oz cans tomato sauce
- 6 bell peppers, halved & seeded
- 1 6-oz can tomato paste
- Salt (to taste)
- Water (as needed)

- 1 12-oz container cottage cheese
- Salt & black pepper, as desired
- ½ tsp oregano
- 2 c each shredded mozzarella and cheddar cheeses

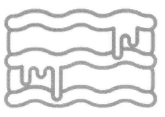

What You'll Do:

1. Preheat oven to 350□F/175□C.
2. After cutting and removing the seeds from the bell peppers, place them on baking sheet- cut side up and sprinkle with salt.
3. Pour ¼ inch/0.64 cm water into pan.
4. Brown ground beef, then drain & discard grease.
5. Add 1 tsp salt, ½ tsp oregano, black pepper, tomato sauce, and tomato paste and bring to a boil.
6. Decrease heat. Simmer for about 15 mins.
7. Layer cottage cheese, mozzarella cheese, cheddar cheese, and meat sauce in each bell pepper.
8. Top with remainder of cheeses.
9. Place in oven and bake for about 50-65 mins.

CHICKEN CACCIATORE

Total Time: 1 h 50 mins | Servings: 6

Nutrition Information: Calories: 513 | Fat: 29 g | Carbs: 11 g | Protein: 50 g | Cholesterol: 149 mg

What You'll Need:

- Whole chicken, cut into quarters
- 2 Tbsp oil
- 1 onion
- 9 oz fresh mushrooms, quartered
- Salt & black pepper, as desired
- 4 cloves garlic, sliced

- 1 tsp oregano
- Red pepper flakes, as desired
- 3 rosemary sprigs
- 1 cup tomato sauce
- ½ c water
- 2 red/2 green bell peppers

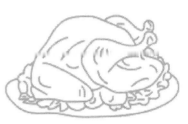

What You'll Do:

1. Preheat oven to 350⬜F/175⬜C. On medium heat, warm olive oil in large Dutch oven.
2. Place chicken in Dutch oven and cook until outside is brown.
3. Then, place into a bowl to catch juices.
4. Add onions & mushrooms and cook until soft (about 5-6 mins).
5. Add salt, black pepper, oregano, rosemary, garlic, tomato sauce, red pepper flakes, and water.
6. Place chicken and juices back in Dutch oven on top of cooked veggies and sprinkle with more salt and black pepper.
7. Top will bell pepper slices.
8. Put lid on the Dutch oven and place in oven- cook for 1 hour 15 mins.

ROAST CHICKEN W/ LEMON & CARROTS

Total Time: 1 h 25 m/Servings: 5

Nutrition Information: Calories: 736 | Fat: 42 g | Carbs: 13 g | Protein: 70 g | Cholesterol: 275 mg

What You'll Need:

- 5 lb/2.26 kg whole chicken
- Salt, to taste
- 1 onion
- 3 Tbsp olive oil
- 1 c light beer

- 1 ½ c chicken broth (more, as needed)
- 6 carrots
- 2 tsp rosemary
- 1 tsp thyme
- 1 lemon

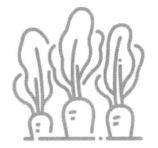

What You'll Do:

1. Preheat oven to 425□F/220□C.
2. Using paper towels, pat chicken dry. Then, cut backbone using kitchen shears.
3. Flip chicken over, breast side up and press down to flatten. Generously season with salt.
4. Over medium heat, warm olive oil in a oven-safe cast iron skillet.
5. Place chicken skin side down and pan fry until golden, approximately 6-7 mins.
6. Transfer to plate, skin side up.
7. Add oil and onion to same skillet and cook until softened, approximately 2-3 mins. Pour beer to skillet to remove any browned bits.
8. Cook until most of the beer is reduced, approximately 2-4 mins.
9. Stir in broth, rosemary, thyme, lemon, and carrots.
10. Place chicken on top of veggies, skin side up.
11. Place in oven and roast until chicken is golden and crispy, approximately 50 mins.
12. Move chicken from pan to platter to rest.
13. Boil broth/juices about 10 mins, until thickened. Serve chicken topped with sauce.

STUFFED SUMMER SQUASH

Total Time: 55 mins | Servings: 5

Nutrition Information: Calories: 148 | Fat: 10 g | Carbs: 6 g | Protein: 8 g | Cholesterol: 24 mg

What You'll Need:

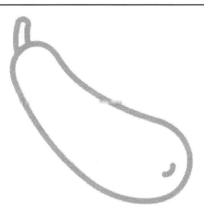

- 2 tsp olive oil
- 4 oz Merguez sausage (remove casing)
- ½ c red bell pepper, diced
- 2 oz crumbled fresh goat cheese
- 5 round summer squash, halved
- Salt & black pepper (to taste)
- 1 Tbsp dry bread crumbs (more, as needed)
- 2 tsp olive oil

What You'll Do:

1. Preheat oven to 375☐F/190☐C.
2. Line baking sheet with foil and coat with 1 tsp olive oil.
3. In nonstick pan over medium heat, add 1 tsp olive oil.
4. Stir in pepper and sausage and cook until sausage is brown and pepper is soft/sweet- about 7-8 mins. Drain off fat.
5. Place sausage mixture and goat cheese in bowl and mix until combined, then set aside.
6. Cut squashes in half and hollow out the centers, then place on baking sheet, cut side up.
7. Fill each with 1-2 Tbsp cheese & sausage mixture. Top with bread crumbs and drizzle with 2 tsp olive oil.
8. Bake until squash is tender and filling is golden, approximately 30 mins.

CANDIED BACON CHICKEN WITH CAULIFLOWER RICE & PECANS

Total Time: 1 h 15 min | Servings: 4

Nutrition Information: Calories: 500 | Fat: 28 g | Carbs: 28 g | Protein: 36 g | Cholesterol: 85 mg

What You'll Need:

- 1/3 c pecans, chopped
- 2 lbs riced cauliflower
- 2 cloves garlic, grated
- 3 Tbsp oil
- 1 Tbsp thyme
- ½ tsp Kosher salt
- Black pepper, to taste
- 4 chicken breasts, sliced thin
- 8 slices bacon
- ¼ c brown sugar
- ¾ tsp chili powder
- ½ c fresh parsley, chopped

What You'll Do:

1. Toast pecans in skillet on medium heat.

2. Preheat oven to 425□F/220□C.

3. Line baking sheet with foil, making sure the foil goes up all sides to catch all juices.

4. In separate bowl, combine cauliflower, 2 tsp thyme, 1 ½ tsp salt, pepper, olive oil, and garlic, and spread on 2/3 of baking sheet. With remainder of thyme, salt, and black pepper, season chicken.

5. Wrap each chicken breast with 2 pieces of bacon, ensuring that chicken is completely covered.

6. Arrange chicken on remaining 1/3 of baking sheet.

7. Mix chili powder and brown sugar in separate bowl and sprinkle half over chicken.

8. Bake for 25 mins.

9. Stir cauliflower and flip chicken. Sprinkle remainder of brown sugar/chili powder mixture over chicken and bake until bacon is crisp and chicken is no longer pink, 20-25 mins. *Your thermometer should read 165□F/74□C when inserted into chicken.* If bacon needs additional crisping, turn oven to broil for a few mins.

10. Remove chicken from baking sheet and stir cauliflower into the drippings.

11. Stir in parsley and toasted pecans. Spoon into bowls and top with chicken.

LETTUCE WRAPS

Total Time: 35 mins | Servings: 4

Nutrition Information: Calories: 388 | Fat: 22 g | Carbs: 24 g | Protein: 23 g | Cholesterol: 69 mg

What You'll Need:

- 16 lettuce leaves
- 1 Tbsp each soy sauce and oil
- 1 lb lean ground beef
- 1 onion, chopped
- ¼ c hoisin sauce
- 2 cloves garlic, minced
- 1 Tbsp rice wine vinegar

- 2 tsp pickled ginger, minced
- Asian chili pepper sauce
- 1 can (8 oz) water chestnuts
- 1 bunch finely chopped green onions
- 2 tsp sesame oil

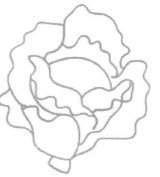

What You'll Do:

1. Rinse lettuce leaves, pat dry, and set aside- take care that you don't tear them.
2. Place skillet on stove and heat on medium-high. Add cooking oil and beef and cook until brown & crumbly, about 5-7 mins. Drain grease and discard.
3. Place beef into separate bowl.
4. In the same skillet, cook onion until tender, about 5-10 mins. Stir in chili pepper sauce, soy sauce, garlic, vinegar, hoisin sauce, and ginger into onions.
5. Add beef, water chestnuts, sesame oil, and green onions. Cook for 2 mins.
6. To serve, pile meat mixture into the center of a serving platter and arrange lettuce leaves around.

BEEF SLAW

Total Time: 31 mins | Servings: 4

Nutrition Information: Calories: 451 | Fat: 28 g | Carbs: 26 | Protein: 25 g | Cholesterol: 70 mg

What You'll Need:

- 1 Tbsp canola oil
- 4 cloves garlic, minced
- 1 Tbsp ginger, minced
- 1 lb ground beef
- 2 heads each white and red cabbage, shredded
- 2 carrots
- 1 red bell pepper

- ½ c soy sauce, reduced sodium
- 2 Tbsp sesame oil
- Dash hot sauce (or more, to taste)
- Salt & black pepper to taste
- 2 Tbsp fresh cilantro, chopped (or more, to taste)
- Lime wedge

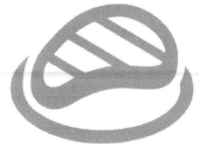

What You'll Do:

1. Heat oil on medium heat in a large skillet/wok.
2. Add garlic & ginger, cook for 2 mins.
3. Add ground beef, cook for 6 mins.
4. Push ground beef to the side in skillet and add the red bell pepper and the shredded white and red cabbage.
5. Mix veggies with beef and cook until veggies are tender, about 5-6 mins.
6. Mix in soy sauce, hot sauce, and sesame oil until well blended.
7. Season with salt & black pepper as desired.

LASAGNA STUFFED MUSHROOMS

Total Time: 50 min | Servings: 2

Nutrition Facts: Calories: 263 | Fat: 12 g | Carbs: 9 g | Protein: 26 g | Cholesterol: 142 mg

What You'll Need:

- ¼ lb ground beef
- ½ c small curd cottage cheese, fat free
- 1 egg
- 1 Tbsp finely chopped green onion
- 1 Tbsp chopped parsley
- Salt & black pepper, to taste
- ¼ pasta sauce
- 6 large mushrooms, stems removed
- ¼ c mozzarella cheese, shredded

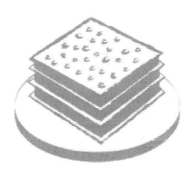

What You'll Do:

1. Preheat oven to 375°F/190°C.
2. Lightly coat baking pan with cooking spray.
3. Place ground beef in skillet and cook for about 10 mins.
4. In a separate bowl, mix salt & pepper, green onion, cottage cheese, parsley, and egg until well blended- add ground beef.
5. Place mushrooms in baking sheet, hollow sides up. Add approximately 1 Tbsp of the filling into each one, allowing remainder to overflow between them.
6. Bake until filling is set, approximately 15 mins.
7. Remove from oven and spread pasta sauce over the top.
8. Sprinkle mozzarella cheese on top of sauce and place back in oven.
9. Broil until cheese is beginning to brown- approximately 5 mins.

SWEET POTATO CARBONARA WITH MUSHROOMS & SPINACH

Total Time: 40 mins | Servings: 5

Nutrition Information: Calories: 312 | Fat: 12 g | Carbs: 38 g | Protein: 15 g | Cholesterol: 130 mg

What You'll Need:

- 2 lbs sweet potatoes
- 3 jumbo eggs
- 1 c grated parmesan cheese
- 1 Tbsp olive oil
- Salt & black pepper, as desired
- 3 strips bacon, chopped
- 1 (8-oz) package mushrooms
- 2 cloves garlic, minced
- 5-oz package baby spinach

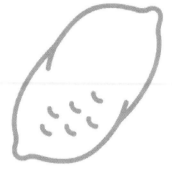

What You'll Do:

1. Bring large pot of water to a boil.
2. Using a julienne veggie peeler or spiralizer, cut sweet potatoes into long, thin strands. You should end up with around 12 cups of noodles.
3. Cook in boiling water, until beginning to soften but not totally tender- should be approximately 1 ½ to 3 mins. Drain, reserving about ¼ c of the water.
4. Place noodles back in pot, off the heat.
5. Combine reserved water, salt, black pepper, eggs, and parmesan cheese in separate bowl. Pour over noodles and toss until coated evenly.
6. Over medium heat, heat oil in skillet.
7. Add bacon & mushrooms, stirring often until liquid has evaporated and mushrooms are beginning to brown.
8. Add garlic, cook for 1 min. Add spinach and cook until wilted.
9. Add veggies to noodles and toss. Top with black pepper.

GRILLED SALMON WRAPS

Total Time: 30 mins | Servings: 4

Nutrition Information: Calories: 306 | Fat: 17 g | Carbs: 7 g | Protein: 28 g | Cholesterol: 79 mg

What You'll Need:

Pico de Gallo:

- 1 tomato, diced and seeded
- ½ red bell pepper, diced and seeded
- ½ red onion, chopped
- Juice from 1 lime

Cream Sauce:

- 2/3 c Greek yogurt, plain
- 2 Tbsp milk, skim
- ½ tsp seasoning blend

Wraps

- 1 lb skinless salmon, grilled and cut into chunks
- 12 radicchio leaves, whole

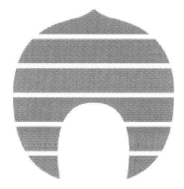

What You'll Do:

1. To make pico de gallo, combine lime juice, red bell pepper, onion, and tomato into small bowl and set aside.

2. In a separate bowl, whisk together seasoning blend, skim milk, and Greek yogurt.

3. Place radicchio leaves on platter and place grilled chunks of salmon on top.

4. Then, top with cream sauce and pico de gallo.

PARMESAN TILAPIA

Total Time: 15 mins | Servings: 8

Nutrition Information: Calories: 224 | Fat: 12 g | Carbs: 0.8 g | Protein: 25 g | Cholesterol: 63 mg

What You'll Need:

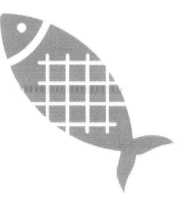

♦ ½ c parmesan cheese

♦ ¼ c softened butter

♦ 3 Tbsp mayo

♦ 2 Tbsp lemon juice

♦ ¼ tsp each dried basil and black pepper

♦ 1/8 tsp each celery salt and onion powder

♦ 2 lbs tilapia fillets

What You'll Do:

1. Preheat oven's broiler and grease broiling pan/line with foil.

2. In small bowl, combine parmesan cheese, lemon juice, mayo, and butter.

3. Season with celery salt, basil, onion powder, and black pepper.

4. Mix thoroughly and set aside.

5. Arrange tilapia fillets on prepared pan.

6. Broil a few inches from heat for 3 mins.

7. Flip fillets and broil for 2 mins.

8. Remove from oven sprinkle parmesan cheese mixture on top.

9. Put fish back in oven and broil until topping is brown/fish is flaky.

PORK CHOPS WITH MUSHROOM SAUCE

Total Time: 40 mins | Servings: 4

Nutrition Information: Calories: 210 | Fat: 8 g | Carbs: 9 g | Protein: 23 g | Cholesterol: 65 mg

What You'll Need:

- 4 pork chops
- Salt & black pepper, as desired
- Garlic salt, as desired
- 1 onion, chopped
- ½ lb sliced mushrooms
- 1 can cream of mushroom soup

What You'll Do:

1. Season chops with garlic salt, black pepper and salt as desired.
2. Place chops in large skillet and brown over medium heat.
3. Add mushrooms and onion, and sauté for 1 min.
4. Pour soup over chops.
5. Cover and reduce temp to med-low.
6. Simmer about 20-30 mins, until chops are tender.

LOW CARB DESSERT RECIPES

ALMOND-RASPBERRY CUPCAKES

Total Prep Time: 40 mins | Servings: 10 cupcakes

Nutrition Information: Calories: 237 | Fat: 20 g | Carbs: 4 g | Protein: 7 g | Fiber: 4 g

What You'll Need:

- 2 large eggs
- ¼ c butter, unsalted
- 1/3 c sweetener of choice
- 1 tsp vanilla extract
- 1 oz water
- ½ tsp fresh squeezed lemon juice

- 2 Tbsp heavy cream
- 2 Tbsp almond extract
- ½ tsp each baking powder & salt
- 2 ½ c almond or coconut flour
- 3 1/3 Tbsp red raspberry preserves, sugar free

What You'll Do:

1. Preheat oven to 350□F/176□C. Place 10 liners in muffin pan and set aside.
2. In small bowl, beat egg yolks with ¼ cup of sweetener, butter, cream, water, lemon juice, and extracts until fully combined and set aside.
3. In medium sized bowl, beat egg whites until frothy. Add remaining 2 Tbsp of sweetener and beat until stiff peaks form. Fold into egg yolk mixture.
4. In a third bowl, mix almond meal, salt, and baking powder.
5. Gently fold into egg mixture before dividing equally between the lined muffin pan.
6. Finally, drop 1 teaspoon of the raspberry jam into the center of each one.
7. Bake for 20 t0 30 mins.
8. Let cool for 20 mins in pan. You can then enjoy these warm or at room temp.
9. Store in fridge for up to one week and serve at room temp. If you want to store longer, place in freezer for up to one month.

CHOCOLATE-PEANUT BUTTER WHIP

Prep Time: 5 mins | Servings: 1

Nutrition Information: Calories: 223 | Fat: 20 g | Carbs: 5 g | Protein: 5 g | Fiber: 3 g

What You'll Need:

- ♦ 1 Tbsp cocoa powder, unsweetened
- ♦ 1 Tbsp natural peanut butter, creamy
- ♦ 2 tsp sweetener of choice
- ♦ 2 Tbsp heavy cream

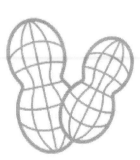

What You'll Do:

1. Blend together cocoa powder, peanut butter, and sweetener.
2. Whip heavy cream, forming soft peaks.
3. Fold whip cream into chocolate peanut butter mix.
4. If desired, use almond butter instead of peanut butter.

PUMPKIN PECAN CHEESECAKE

Prep Time: 1 hr 15 mins | Servings: 8

Nutrition Information: Calories: 488 | Fat: 47 g | Carbs: 7 g | Protein: 10 g | Fiber: 3 g

What You'll Need:

Crust:

♦ 1 ½ c pecan halves

♦ 1 Tbsp sweetener

♦ ½ tsp cinnamon

♦ 2 Tbsp butter, unsalted

♦ 1 large egg white

Filling:

♦ 2 blocks (12-Oz each) of cream cheese

♦ 2/3 c sweetener

♦ 1 c heavy cream

♦ 15 oz canned pumpkin, no salt

♦ 1 tsp each pumpkin pie spice and vanilla extract

♦ 3 large eggs, whole

What You'll Do:

Crust:

1. Preheat oven to 350F/176C.

2. In blender/food processor, combine pecans, 1 Tbsp sweetener, and cinnamon and process until finely ground and mixed well.

3. Add melted butter and egg white and blend just enough to combine.

4. Press mixture into 9" springform pan and bake until golden- about 8-10 mins.

5. Allow to cool on wire rack.

Filling:

1. Decrease oven temp to 325F/162C.

2. In a large bowl, combine cream, cream cheese, and 2/3 c sweetener, using electric mixer to blend until smooth.

3. Add canned pumpkin, pumpkin pie spice, and vanilla, mixing well.

4. Beat eggs in one at a time, until just combined.

5. Pour batter into crust and bake until just set- about 45-50 mins.

6. Turn oven off and allow pie to stand for 10 mins.

7. Move to wire rack and cool completely. Cover and put in fridge until chilled. Slice and serve.

VANILLA ALMOND BUTTER COOKIES

Nutrition Information: Calories: 55 | Fat: 4 g | Protein:2 g | Carbs: 2 g | Fiber: 0.7 g

What You'll Need:

- 1 ½ c almonds, slivered and blanched
- ¾ c soy flour, whole grain
- 3 Tbsp baking powder
- ¾ c sweetener
- 1 large whole egg & 1 large egg yolk
- 2 Tbsp vanilla extract
- ¼ c butter, unsalted

What You'll Do:

1. Preheat oven to 375☐F/190☐C.
2. In blender/food processor, finely grind almonds and mix with soy flour, sweetener, and baking powder.
3. In separate bowl, on medium speed, mix whole egg, butter, egg yolk, and vanilla. Mixture will not be smooth.
4. Fold in soy flour mixture with rubber spatula until combined.
5. Form 24 small balls with dough and place on ungreased baking sheet.
6. Using a fork, slightly flatten to silver dollar size.
7. Bake 8-10 mins and allow to cool on baking sheets before moving to wire rack.

TIRAMISU CUPCAKES

Total Prep Time: 40 mins | Servings: 6

Nutrition Information: Calories: 293 | Fat: 24 g | Carbs: 3 g | Protein: 5 g | Fiber: 11 g

What You'll Need:

- 3 Tbsp butter, unsalted
- 3 large whole eggs
- ¼ c sucralose sweetener
- 5 Tbsp xylitol sweetener
- 4 Tbsp vanilla extract
- ¼ c coconut flour, organic & high fiber
- ¼ tsp baking powder
- ¼ tsp salt
- 4 oz mascarpone
- 1 ¼ Tbsp instant coffee powder
- ½ c heavy cream
- ½ oz water

What You'll Do:

NOTE: This recipe uses both sucralose and xylitol sweetener to give a rounded sweetness.

Cupcakes:

1. Preheat oven to 375°F/190°C. Place liners in muffin tin and set aside.
2. With an electric mixer, blend sucralose sweetener and butter until fluffy- about 2 mins.
3. Add eggs, 1 tsp vanilla, baking powder, salt, and coconut flour, blending until smooth. Divide batter between 6 muffin cups.
4. Bake for about 15 mins.
5. Let rest in pan for 5 mins before removing to place on cooling rack.

Soaking syrup:

1. Combine 1 tsp instant coffee, 1 ½ Tbsp water, 2 Tbsp xylitol, and 2 tsp vanilla.
2. Poke cupcakes with toothpick and pour soaking syrup over each one.

Mascarpone Frosting:

1. Blend mascarpone cheese, ¼ instant coffee, 1 tsp vanilla, and 3 Tbsp xylitol until smooth.
2. In separate bowl, whip heavy cream until stiff peaks form.
3. Fold mascarpone cheese mixture into whipped cream until combined.
4. Place mixture in decorator/pastry bag with a fancy tip (if desired) and pipe onto cooled cupcakes- or you can just spread frosting onto cupcakes if you prefer.
5. Serve at room temp, dusted with cocoa powder. May be kept in fridge overnight in airtight container, if desired.

LOW CARB SNACK RECIPES

BLACKBERRY-COCONUT FAT BOMBS

Total Prep Time: 10 mins | Servings: 16 bite-size squares

Nutrition Information: Calories: 170 | Fat: 18 g | Carbs: 3 g | Protein: 1 g

What You'll Need:

- 1 c coconut butter
- 1 c coconut oil
- ½ c blackberries, strawberries, or raspberries
- ½ tsp sweetener, more to taste
- ½ tsp vanilla extract (or ¼ tsp vanilla powder)
- 1 Tbsp lemon juice

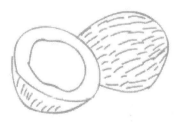

What You'll Do:

1. Place coconut oil & butter (& if frozen, berries) in pot. Heat until just combined on medium heat. If using fresh berries, do not add them yet.

2. Place oil mixture and other ingredients into blender and blend. You must ensure that oil mixture is not too hot, otherwise separation will occur.

3. Using parchment paper, line square pan and pour mixture in.

4. Place in fridge for an hour or until mixture has hardened.

5. Cut into squares and enjoy.

6. Store in fridge, covered.

PIZZA BITES

Total Prep Time: 25 mins | Servings: 28

Nutrition Information: Calories: 60 | Fat: 5 g | Carbs: 1 | Protein: 2.5 g

What You'll Need:

- ½ c almond flour
- ½ c parmesan cheese, grated
- ½ tsp each basil and garlic powder
- ¼ tsp each salt, oregano, and thyme
- ¼ c coconut flour
- 2 tsp baking powder
- 4-oz mozzarella, shredded
- 2 to 3 oz chopped pepperoni
- 4 Tbsp butter, room temp
- 2 large eggs
- ½ c sour cream

Other Ingredients (as desired)

- ¼ c olives, chopped
- ½ bell pepper or small onion, chopped and sautéed
- 4 oz mushrooms, chopped and sautéed
- If you wish, omit basil, oregano, and thyme
- and use 1 tsp Italian seasoning instead

What You'll Do:

1. Preheat oven to 350☐F/176☐C. Place parchment paper on 2 pans and set aside.
2. In a medium-size bowl, add dry ingredients and blend.
3. Add the rest of the ingredients and mix until well blended with a spatula or wooden spoon.
4. Use a small scoop for smaller bites and a medium scoop for larger bites to measure dough onto pans and place 3 inches apart.
5. Bake until brown, 15-20 mins.
6. Serve with pizza sauce or ranch dressing.

SALT & VINEGAR ZUCCHINI CHIPS

Total Prep Time: 12 hours 15 mins | Servings: 8

Nutrition Information: Calories: 40 | Fat: 3 g | Carbs: 3 g | Protein: .7 g

What You'll Need:

- 2-3 medium zucchini, thinly sliced
- 2 Tbsp olive oil, sunflower oil, or avocado oil
- 2 Tbsp white balsamic vinegar
- 2 tsp sea salt

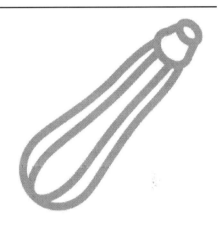

What You'll Do:

1. Slice zucchini thin.
2. Combine oil and vinegar in a separate bowl.
3. Place zucchini in bowl with oil & vinegar and toss until covered.
4. Place zucchini in even layers in food dehydrator and sprinkle with sea salt. Depending upon how thin your zucchini is and your dehydrator, the time will vary- from 8 to 14 hours.
5. These can be done in your oven if you do not have a food dehydrator.
6. Using parchment paper, line baking sheet and place zucchini in an even layer.
7. Bake at 200□F/93□C for 2-3 hours, flipping chips over halfway through cook time.
8. Must be stored in a container with a tight seal.

CHOCOLATE QUINOA BITES

Total Prep Time: 10 mins | Servings: 12

Nutrition Facts: Calories: 175 | Fat: 13 g | Carbs: 13 g | Protein: 3 g

What You'll Need:

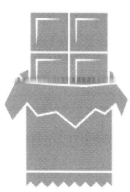

- ¼ c coconut oil
- ¼ c maple syrup
- 1/3 c unsweetened cocoa powder
- ½ c nut/seed butter of choice
- ½ c quinoa, cooked
- ½ c quinoa flakes
- ½ c coconut flakes
- Sea salt for sprinkling, if desired

What You'll Do:

1. Line baking sheet with parchment paper.
2. Melt coconut oil, syrup, and cocoa powder together in small saucepan over medium heat, whisking until combined.
3. Add almond butter. Blend until smooth.
4. Remove from heat and fold in coconut flakes, quinoa, and quinoa flakes.
5. Using a cookie scoop, drop onto prepared baking sheet, and sprinkle with sea salt (if desired) and place in freezer for about 30 minutes to set.
6. For best results, store in freezer in airtight container- but can be kept in fridge, if you want a softer consistency.

PEPPER NACHOS

Total Prep Time: 20 mins | Servings: 6

Nutrition Information: Calories: 351 | Cholesterol: 96 mg | Fat: 21 g | Carbs: 6 g | Protein: 28 g

What You'll Need:

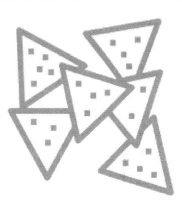

- 1 tsp each garlic powder, cumin, and paprika
- 1 Tbsp chili powder
- ½ tsp each salt, pepper, and oregano
- ¼ tsp red pepper flakes (more if you want it hotter)
- 1 lb ground beef
- 1 lb mini peppers, halved & seeded
- 1 ½ c cheddar cheese, shredded
- ½ c tomato, chopped
- Other toppings, such as
- avocado, olives, chopped jalapenos, sour cream, etc.

What You'll Do:

1. Combine all spices in separate bowl and set aside.
2. Brown beef in skillet over medium heat- about 7-10 mins. Add spice mixture and sauté until combined.
3. Preheat oven to 400□F/204□C and line baking sheet with parchment paper or foil.
4. Arrange peppers close together, cut side up, in a single layer.
5. Sprinkle with ground beef and shredded cheese, making sure each pepper has some on it.
6. Bake 5-10 mins.
7. Take out of oven and add extra toppings as desired.

LOW CARB SMOOTHIE RECIPES

CHOCOLATE-AVOCADO SMOOTHIE

Prep Time: 5 mins | Servings: 1

Nutrition Information: Calories: 582 | Cholesterol: 81 mg | Carbs: 30 g | Protein: 9 g

What You'll Need:

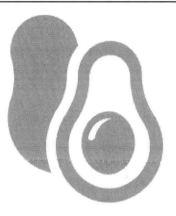

- Avocado, peel & remove pit
- ½ c heavy cream (decrease calorie count by substituting milk)
- 1 Tbsp dark cocoa powder
- 3 tsp Splenda (or preferred sweetener)
- 1 c water

What You'll Do:

1. Place all ingredients in blender and blend until smooth.
2. Serve cold.

VERY BERRY SMOOTHIE

Prep Time: 5 mins | Servings: 1

Nutrition Information: Calories: 129 | Fat: 3 g | Cholesterol: 7 mg | Carbs: 18 g | Protein: 7 g

What You'll Need:

♦ ½ c unsweetened almond milk

♦ ½ c low-fat yogurt

♦ ½ cup frozen berry mix (blackberries, raspberries, strawberries, blueberries)

♦ 1 tsp sweetener of choice

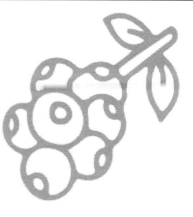

What You'll Do:

1. Place all ingredients in blender and blend until smooth.

2. Serve cold.

CHOCOLATE PEANUT BUTTER SMOOTHIE

Prep Time: 5 mins | Servings: 1

Nutrition Information: Calories: 457 | Total Fat: 32 g |Cholesterol: 85 mg | Total Carbs: 20 g | Protein: 25 g

What You'll Need:

- 1 c almond milk, unsweetened
- 2 c ice
- 2 Tbsp natural peanut butter, unsweetened
- 2 Tbsp cocoa powder, unsweetened
- 1 scoop vanilla flavored protein powder
- 2 Tbsp heavy whipping cream
- ¼ tsp vanilla extract
- Sweetener, to taste (optional)

What You'll Do:

1. Place almond milk, whipping cream, peanut butter, vanilla extract, cocoa powder, protein powder, and sweetener into blender.
2. Blend until smooth and serve cold.

COFFEE SMOOTHIE

Prep Time: 5 mins | Servings: 1

Nutrition Information: Calories: 294 | Fat: 19 g | Cholesterol: 91 mg | Carbs: 10 g | Protein: 23 g

What You'll Need:

- ♦ 16 oz vanilla flavored almond milk, unsweetened
- ♦ 1 tsp instant coffee
- ♦ 1 Tbsp ground flax seed
- ♦ 2 Tbsp cream cheese
- ♦ 1 scoop protein powder

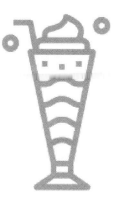

What You'll Do:

1. Place all ingredients in blender and blend until smooth.
2. Serve immediately.

AVOCADO/SPINACH/STRAWBERRY SMOOTHIE

Prep Time: 5 mins | Servings: 1

Nutrition Information: Calories: 296 | Fat: 22 g | Cholesterol 0 mg | Carbs: 26 g | Protein: 5 g

What You'll Need:

- 1 medium avocado
- ½ c frozen sliced strawberries
- 4 oz grape juice
- ½ cup fresh spinach

What You'll Do:

1. Place all ingredients in blender and blend until smooth.

Bonus:
10 Ways to Lose Weight Fast

These days, it seems like everywhere you look, there's someone that's looking for the secret to lose weight fast. While there's no magical solution, the best thing to do is to stop the yo-yo dieting and commit to a true lifestyle change- such as the low-carb lifestyle. After all, most diets require you to restrict yourself and are not realistic solutions. In this section, we'll outline 10 ways that you can jump start weight loss as you begin your journey.

Begin Your Day with Warm Lemon Water

Lemon water will get your digestive system moving and help flush out toxins. You'll also want to commit to drinking at least 8 glasses of water every day. This will help speed up your metabolism and curb your hunger.

Get at least 30 mins of Physical Activity Daily

Exercising will not only help you lose weight, but also help you maintain your weight. Plus, when you work up a sweat, your body is able to fight off a variety of health conditions/disease- and your mood is improved. Just because you're committing to working out doesn't mean that you're stuck to the gym. There are lots of ways that you can burn calories. Find a few things you enjoy and start practicing them. You might want to consider alternating them as well, so you don't get burnt out.

Be Sure to Get Your Fiber

Foods that are rich in fiber keep you feeling fuller longer. This means you won't eat as much. In addition, fiber aids in digestion and lowers your blood sugar and cholesterol.

Consume Healthy Protein Sources at Every Meal

Protein also keeps you feeling fuller longer, as well as promoting muscle growth and repair. However, you must make sure that you're consuming clean proteins, such as pastured eggs, organic chicken, wild salmon, or grass-fed beef. If you're a vegan, consider adding healthy grains/beans and flax, hemp, and chia seeds.

Pay Attention to What You're Eating

Make sure that you pay attention to what you're eating and what is actually going to give you nourishment. If there's not a good reason behind eating something, you probably shouldn't be eating it. Don't eat while you're distracted- and take it slow because it takes about 20 mins from the time you begin your meal for your brain to realize that your stomach is full.

Choose Healthy Snacks

Choosing healthy snacks is just as important as choosing healthy meals because they help balance your blood sugar and energy levels. You shouldn't worry about snacks labeled diet/low fat/fat free. The idea is to choose fresh, whole foods.

Discover Healthy Alternatives to Your Favorite Treats

If there is something that you really enjoy, don't eliminate it from your diet. Instead, give yourself permission to splurge once a week- but take the time to make it yourself. This way, you have control of what goes into it. Unfortunately, it's easy to find unhealthy recipes, so it will take a little effort to find some healthier alternatives.

Learn to Manage Your Stress

Cortisol, which is the hormone that is related to stress, results in belly fat, food cravings, and increased appetite. Take the time to de-stress when you feel it coming on. This can be by writing in a journal, practicing yoga/meditation, practicing deep breathing exercises, and many other activities. Everyone is faced with stress. The key is learning the best way for you to deal with it.

Kick Those Bad Habits

Of course, reaching that ideal, healthy lifestyle is not just about changing your eating habits. There are many other things that could be sabotaging your life: smoking, drinking too much soda or alcohol, not getting enough sleep, and much more. Take an inventory of your daily habits and start changing those that you think are holding you back. This is going to be difficult, so take baby steps.

Make a Plan to be Successful

Every successful person started with a plan in place to encourage that success. If you don't plan to succeed, then you're planning to fail. If you will make an effort to remove all unhealthy foods from you kitchen and you start making meal prep a priority, you'll find that it's easier to be committed to your goals.

While it's true that dieting will jumpstart your weight loss journey, you have to make an effort to lose and maintain it. The best thing to do is to make some changes in your lifestyle and soon, you'll find that the extra weight is gone and you're feeling much better in all aspects: physically, mentally, and emotionally. If you do slip back into your old habits, don't beat yourself up- just reaffirm your commitment to changing your life. Good luck!

Disclaimer

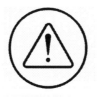

The opinions and ideas of the author contained in this publication are designed to educate the reader in an informative and helpful manner. While we accept that the instructions will not suit every reader, it is only to be expected that the recipes might not gel with everyone. Use the book responsibly and at your own risk. This work with all its contents, does not guarantee correctness, completion, quality or correctness of the provided information. Always check with your medical practitioner should you be unsure whether to follow a low carb eating plan. Misinformation or misprints cannot be completely eliminated. Human error is real!

Cover design: oliviaprodesign

Cover photo: zarzamora / shutterstock.com